D1784081

Understanding
Rheumatism

F. Dudley Hart
MD, FRCP

This is a Family Doctor booklet published by the British
Medical Association, BMA House, Tavistock Square, London WC1H 9JR

Contents

What is rheumatism?   3

Aches, pains and strains—the simple ones   5

Aches and pains—the not so simple ones   10

Some arthritic disorders   15

Things that help—and things that don't   23

Living with rheumatism   27

We are indebted to the Arthritis and Rheumatism Council for their kind permission to use the brilliant illustrations by the late Leslie Starke

Editor: Norma Pearce
Medical Editor: Tony Smith, MA BM BCh
ISBN: 0 7279 0188 5

What is rheumatism?

Rheumatism is a term used so loosely that really all it usually means is "aches and pains and possibly stiffness in muscles, bones, ligaments, and joints anywhere in the body". In other words not arising from heart, lungs, intestines, and other structures *inside* the body.

These aches and pains may be due to a large number of conditions ranging from a simple sprained ankle to a severe rheumatoid arthritis, and defined thus all of us have "rheumatism" at some time in our lives. Unpleasant, annoying, and tedious though it may be, it is only rarely serious and very seldom affects general health or alters one's insurance policy. Arthritis on the other hand means inflammation of one or several joints. This again can be due to many conditions ranging from German measles to rheumatoid arthritis. The term arthrosis describes a condition primarily due to degenerative (wear and tear) rather than inflammatory changes in a joint.

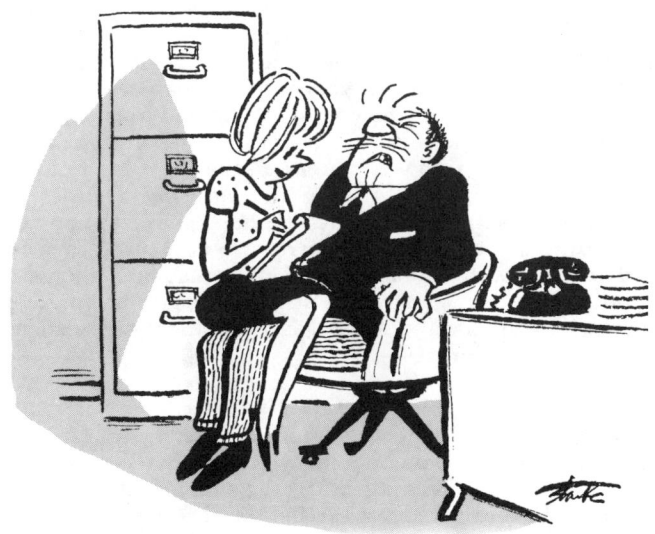

Osteoarthrosis commonly affects weight bearing joints—the knee in particular

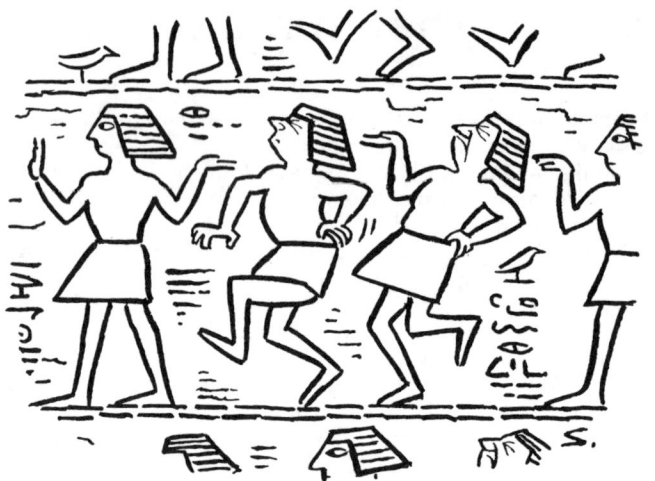

Backaches and disc trouble have been a curse to mankind since ancient days

How did the word rheumatism arise? In ancient times it was thought that these unpleasant aches and pains were caused by one of the four cardinal "humours" discharged from the blood into the muscles and joints. "Rheum" in both ancient Latin and Greek, meant a flow of watery discharge, a kind of ugly catarrh flowing into the tissues and carrying disease into them. This, in fact, certainly does not happen except in a very few conditions such as gout, where uric acid may leave the blood and crystallise out in the joints causing agonising discomfort, but in rheumatoid arthritis there may be an excess of fluid in the inflamed joints and surrounding tissues causing stiffness and swelling.

Rheumatism—an "umbrella" word

The word "rheumatism" therefore means very little. Any ache or pain in muscle, bone, or joint which cannot be explained tends to be called "rheumatism" by the sufferer, or sometimes "fibrositis" under the impression that the fibrous or connective tissue becomes inflamed, which is rarely the case. So if the words "aches and pains" were used he would be saying the same thing but would be stating a fact instead of implying a disease. **Rheumatic fever,** however, *is* a definite disease and can be a serious one, particularly in childhood. Happily it is now a rarity here but 40 and more years ago it was the commonest cause of heart disease under the age of 16.

Aches, pains, and strains

—The simple ones

Let us start with **leg cramps**. If these are in the calf muscles, come on after walking a certain distance, go off with rest, and reappear after walking the same distance they are important, for they may well be due to thickening of the arteries of the legs and should be reported to the sufferer's doctor. If, however, they come on at night, affect any muscles in either leg, and even if they are severe and wake you up they are unpleasant but *not* important or serious in terms of general health.

Cramps at night

In cramp the muscles bunch up and can be felt as hard firm lumps: massaging them, getting out of bed, and standing or moving the limbs will rapidly bring relief and the painful hard muscular contractions will quickly disappear. Those prone to muscle spasms often take a tablet of quinine on retiring to prevent them occurring and say it helps greatly, though how or why is uncertain. Some folk with bad varicose veins often suffer cramps and find that sleeping with the foot of the bed raised a foot or so lessens or prevents them. Night cramps are extremely common and usually occur in healthy people of any age, even children and teenagers.

Calf cramps which come on during the day after walking (as already mentioned) usually occur in men over 45 and are important. They should not be confused with pains in other muscles, however; such as thigh, knee, ankle, and feet, which may come on with any exertion and are often due to osteo-arthrosis.

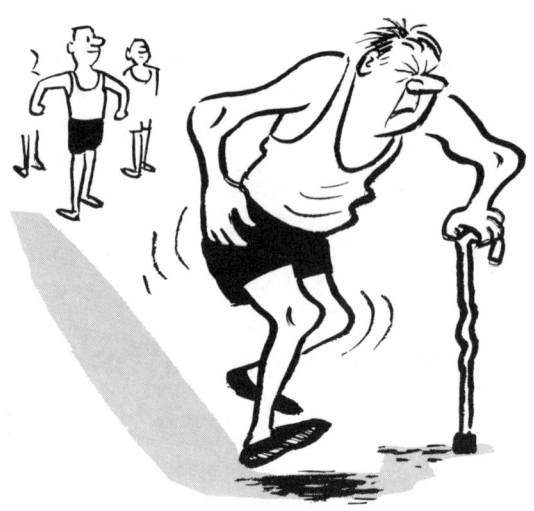

In active rheumatoid arthritis it is of no help to "try and walk it off"

"Growing pains"

While the process of growing is not itself a cause, aches and pains in the arms and legs in growing children are quite common, particularly in legs. Most of them are not due to serious disease. The mother of 40 years and more ago always feared that they might be due to rheumatic fever, and the mother of today fears that some type of rheumatic condition may be affecting her child.

Most growing pains are *not* due to arthritis and rheumatic fever is very uncommon in this country today. Strain, fatigue, low grade ill-health, badly fitting shoes or boots, dislike of going to school—101 things may cause these pains, and rapidly growing, tall children (often of tall parents) seem more prone than others. If swelling of the knees occurs (so called water on the knees) arthritis may well be present but in most children with growing pains there is no swelling, just aches, which will pass as the child grows up.

Creaking, cracking, and clicking joints

Some young people can produce the most horrific clicks and snapping noises by bending their fingers, toes, and other joints (they do it on request as a kind of party trick). These castanet sounds or calypso like noises are not at all serious and do *not* mean that the "musician" will later be an arthritic cripple. "Double jointed" people, however, who can bend their joints much further than normal people, are more liable to suffer strains and sprains, are more likely to experience joint pains than most of us less elastic people, and can also injure their joints more readily.

In later life, past the age of 30 to 40, cracking noises increase in knees, feet, neck, and shoulders particularly and become audible to most people. Going downstairs may become quite a musical experience as one grows older but such clicks, creaks, and cracks are routine accompaniments of middle age and have no awful significance. Grating joints in the knee caps or across the back of the neck can be felt with the hands and can often be heard: again these are not a sign of disease but of the fact that one is growing a little older and more mature! Solitary cracks and clonks may be experienced at any age in almost any joint. These are normal and not a sign of disease.

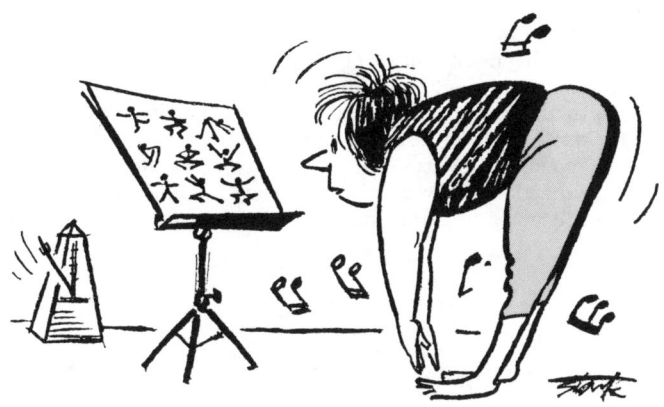

A calypso of clicks and creaks does not mean the "musician" will later be crippled with osteoarthrosis

Pins and needles

Pins and needles, common in the hands and arms, are not usually due to arthritis but can be caused by pressure on a nerve—by lying on one arm in deep sleep, by hanging an arm over a chair back which presses on the nerves in the armpit, or by using a crutch in the same way pressing up under the shoulder. The median nerve may be compressed at the wrist and cause tingling and pins and needles sensations up the arm, worse at night and often interfering with sleep. Nerve compression may follow a fracture or dislocation of the wrist but in women may occur at the menopause without any injury. More rarely it may be due to early rheumatoid arthritis, thyroid deficiency, or some other disorder. Sensations of pins and needles which come on only occasionally in hands and arms or feet and legs and last only a short while are almost certainly of no importance but if they persist and are troublesome for days or weeks tell your doctor about them.

Unpleasant pricking sensations in the bases of the thumbs where they meet the wrists are an early sign of osteoarthrosis of this joint. This is an unpleasant but not serious affliction which does not affect general health and is usually only a painful nasty nuisance.

Stiff neck

An acute stiff neck may come on suddenly—often after a draught through a car window, after a long drive, or after sleeping with the neck bent sideways. Painful stiff necks usually settle in a few hours or days with heat (a warm scarf or well wrapped hot water bottle often helps), rest, and pain relieving drugs. If they persist, massage or neck traction and very gentle manipulation may cure the condition. A chroni-

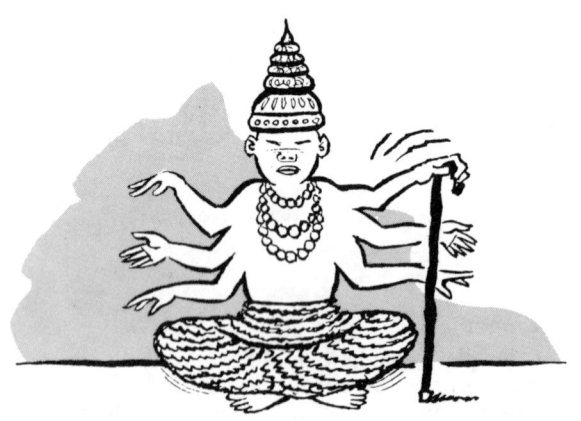

Stiff necks can be brought on by unusual activity

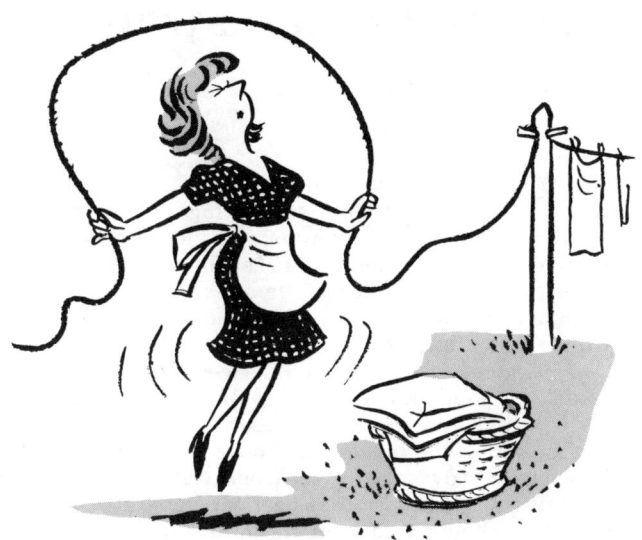

To fight any illness successfully it is essential to keep as fit as possible

cally stiff neck may be due to an old injury or to osteoarthrosis, for in late middle age the cartilaginous discs between the vertebrae narrow and become less elastic and the neck stiffens. Changes which can be seen on an *x*-ray, especially in the lower neck, are almost always present after the age of 60, even if symptoms are slight.

Other more rare arthritic conditions, such as ankylosing spondylitis, (see page 18) come on much earlier in life, more often in men than women. In general arthritis is a relatively rare cause of stiffness of the neck at any age whereas osteoarthrosis, or disc or joint degeneration (so called cervical spondylosis) is common after middle age. In old age stiffness is usually *not* accompanied by much pain.

Aches, pains, and strains

—The not so simple ones

Scattered throughout the body are small, soft, fluid containing bursae (*bursa* is Latin for purse), acting as soft cushions between bones and muscles, diminishing friction, and making for smooth movements. There are 156 such bursae in the body. Usually people are unaware of their existence but if they become inflamed and swollen they produce symptoms and the condition is called **bursitis**.

This may happen as a result of excessive friction as in housemaid's or nun's knee, when swellings appear over the front of this joint as a result of excessive kneeling. Student's elbow or boozer's elbow may result from prolonged pressure on the elbow, bunions over the big toe from pressure of shoes, and so on. Bursitis may also occur as part of a generalised disease such as gout or rheumatoid arthritis but in most cases it is just due to repeated local friction and recovers satisfactorily when the local pressures are removed.

Frozen shoulder

The shoulder is a highly mobile joint with a very large range of movements. Just as the essence of the hip joint is *stability* so the particular attribute of the shoulder is *mobility*. Here tendons cross the joint in close proximity to a bursa (the subacromial bursa) which acts as a protective cushion beneath the bone. If any inflammatory process starts up in the area the various structures become painful on movement and adhere to one another, so that the painful shoulder becomes in time the frozen shoulder, which cannot be moved because of stiffness rather than pain. In most cases, happily, as soon as the pain abates normal movements can be performed again showing that the shoulder was not truly frozen, only painful.

A painful stiff shoulder may occur as a result of arthritis of the shoulder joint but more frequently occurs as a result of inflammatory changes *around* the joint, the so called peri-arthritis. Violent manipulations and movements may make such joints worse by tearing tissues which are adherent to each other, an example being the "check-rein shoulder" when a horse, being reined in or checked by the coach or cab driver would throw its head forward and by suddenly pulling on the reins tear the driver's shoulder capsule. Such frozen shoulders rarely come to harm with simple exercises done by the patient himself but they can often be aggravated by vigorous movement done by others.

Tennis elbow and golfer's elbow

Tennis elbow is a condition where a small area at the muscle insertion into the bone on the outer side of the elbow becomes acutely painful and tender, as a result of a small tear often from vigorous back-handed strokes on the tennis court, sometimes from other injuries to the area, sometimes for no apparent reason. Such a condition (like the frozen shoulder) is often worsened by further exertions which aggravate the lesion starting the whole thing up again.

Golfer's elbow is a similar but usually milder condition affecting the inner side of the elbow. Injections of local anaesthetic and hydrocortisone often help greatly in both cases but may cause severe pain initially for 24 hours or more. The elbow lesions may sometimes last for many months whatever is done. Vigorous use, as with the frozen shoulder, often worsens the condition.

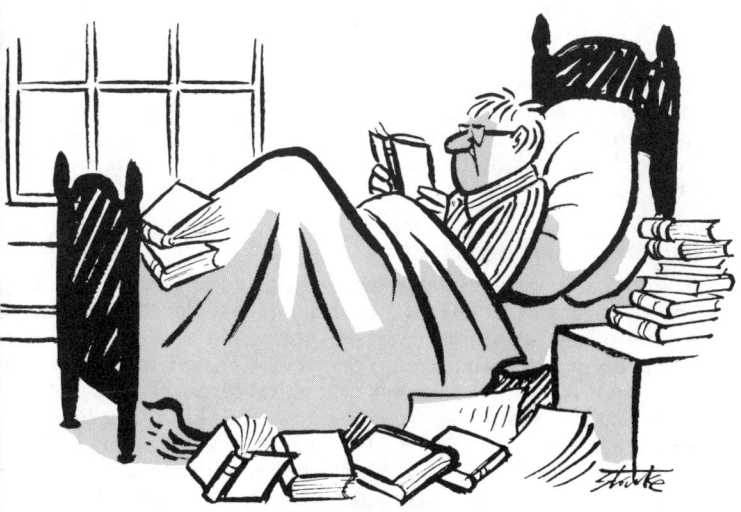

It is not a good thing to retire to bed and stay there in any form of rheumatism or arthritis

Water on the knee

The knee has several bursae around it and one at the back of the knee (Baker's cyst) usually communicates with the knee joint and thus may act as an overflow tank when the knee becomes over full of fluid as a result of injury, excessive exercise or strain, or actual arthritis. A bulge on the back of the knee may therefore be nature's way of easing the fluid pressure in a knee joint by taking the overflow.

What is fibrositis?

This is still a popular term but is no longer used by doctors as the idea that these pains are due to an acute inflammation of the fibrous tissue under the skin and in the muscles has been given up for lack of good evidence of its existence. Sufferers of "fibrositis" usually mean aches and pains across neck and shoulders and upper back. These can be due to almost anything in the medical dictionary but are often caused by pain referred from the neck and spine due to strains, minor injuries, and areas of degeneration in bone and cartilage.

There are many other causes such as fatigue, prolonged bad posture, depression, anxiety, or combinations of these. Your shoulder muscles ache when you have a fever and even a TAB innoculation against typhoid may cause such an ache for a day or two. Undue exertions especially when "out of training" may produce severe "fibrositis" next day. Aches and crackles round and under the shoulder blades and upper back are common and can be very tedious and unpleasant but happily do not reflect any serious underlying disorder, and the so called "fibrous nodules" are just innocent lumps of fat or fibrous tissue, or both.

Neuritis or neuralgia

Neuritis or neuralgia is due to irritation of or pressure on a nerve and is characterised by pins and needles, pains, and various other sensations referred down the arm or leg, an example being **sciatica** from pressure of a lumbar disc on a nerve root. A most unpleasant type is **trigeminal neuralgia** where extreme pain is felt in one cheek, the skin being left so sensitive that even wiping the face with a towel is agonisingly painful. **Shingles** is due to actual inflammation of the nerve by a virus, the pain appearing as a nasty pricking burning sensation in the skin a day or two before the typical rash appears.

Hands in trouble

Hands thicken as they grow older, particularly round the end joints of the fingers. This is due to a thickening and strengthening of bone around an aging cartilage (see Osteoarthrosis). A thickening of the palms of the hands, more common in men than women, is called **Dupuytren's contraction** after the famous French surgeon who first described it. This thickening in the palmar tissues under the skin may lead to contraction of the finger which sometimes calls for surgery, not for pain as the condition is painless, but because function of the hand becomes impaired.

Lumps and bumps

Ganglia, small semi-solid lumps which sometimes occur on the backs of wrists, are painless and of little consequence. The old fashioned, do it yourself treatment was to bang them hard with a large heavy book (the Bible was usually recommended) but they are innocent lumps and are best left alone. Very rarely they may be an early sign of rheumatoid arthritis.

Feet and ankles

Many deformities are caused by the silly shoes we wear. Ladies are more guilty than men in this respect, and in the pursuit of elegance will cram their feet into pointed shoes then elevate the heel so that all five toes are pushed forward into an area large enough to accommodate only two or three.

This leads to the big toe being pushed sideways towards the middle toe, and the other toes are rearranged around the middle one, some being displaced backwards. As a result, painful hard areas form in the skin from friction of the toes on the shoe above. The natural shape of the foot can be best seen in those who have never worn shoes. As the big toe is pushed sideways its base suffers more friction on the shoe and an inflamed area or bunion may develop. High heels may cause friction in the Achilles tendon running into the back of the heel.

Another common complaint is swelling of ankles and feet, again more common in women than men. Although swelling may in some cases be caused by heart or kidney disease or to arthritis in foot or ankle, far more common causes are prolonged immobility in standing or sitting positions (to be avoided as much as possible) and varicose veins.

The patient often attributes this problem to "poor circulation" and in a sense this is partly correct. The heart's action pumps blood out to the tissues through the arteries but the return from the tissues to the heart from the legs is partly from muscular activity in the legs, the muscular tone of the veins, and gravity. In a sense we are all buckets of blood, our veins in the erect position being full up to our Adam's apple or top of the sternum or breastbone. Congested veins in your hands or feet empty immediately they are elevated above this level.

Keep moving

Sitting still for prolonged periods, as in long car or aeroplane trips, often therefore produces swelling of the feet and ankles as was seen often in severe degree in the blitz in the last war when many thousands of Londoners had to sit up all night in air raid shelters, often in cramped conditions.

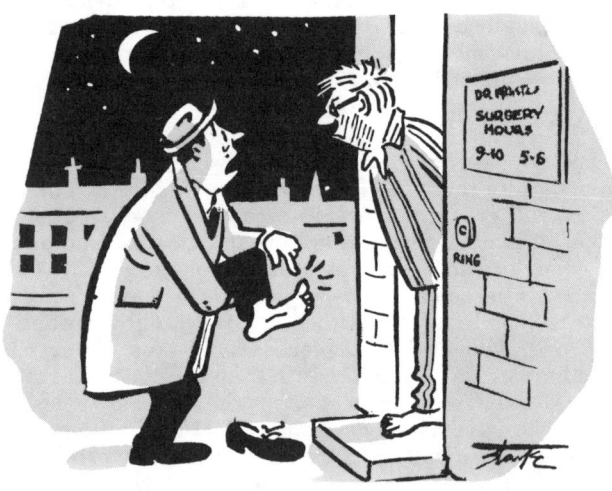

In gout, the earlier you start treatment the better but it can wait until the morning surgery!

Some arthritic disorders

Arthritis literally means inflammation of a joint or joints, rather than one specific condition and will therefore be dealt with under separate headings.

Osteoarthrosis (osteoarthritis)

In this condition, although some inflammatory changes are present for some of the time, the essential changes are degenerative, ie coming on gradually over a period of time. Our young growing cartilages, which act as firm elastic washers, pads, or shock absorbers between the bones, start aging in the mid-20s, losing some of their springy elasticity very gradually and slowly as the years go by. By the time we are in our 50s and 60s some of our cartilages are narrowed to some extent and aches and pains may be noticed in those areas, the commonest being the finger tip joints, the thumb bases at the wrist, the lower part of the back of the neck and the lower back, the big toe joints, and also the knee joints.

In the process the bones each side of the wearing cartilage often thicken and become stronger but stiffer and rather unsightly and sometimes, but only sometimes, they may ache and become painful. Repeated small injuries play a part, particularly in the finger joint and the big toe (the weight bearing joint which suffers most minor insults, not least being the wearing of unsatisfactory shoes) and the hard working hand may show more thickening than the one unused to daily and repeated physical minor knocks.

The two areas in the spine most affected by degenerative changes are the base of the neck and the lower lumbar spine (the lumbago area). These areas, though almost always suffering some degenerative changes as the years advance, are only occasionally painful and rarely severely so. The change from the supple sapling of 19 to the gnarled oak of 70 years is a very gradual one and, happily, only occasionally severely painful.

Knees and hips

Osteoarthrotic knees and hips that are severely affected can, however, be a considerable disability. Previous injuries or congenital abnormalities can predispose to osteoarthrosis if the bones are out of proper alignment. It rarely affects wrists, elbows, or shoulders unless previously injured. The disorder

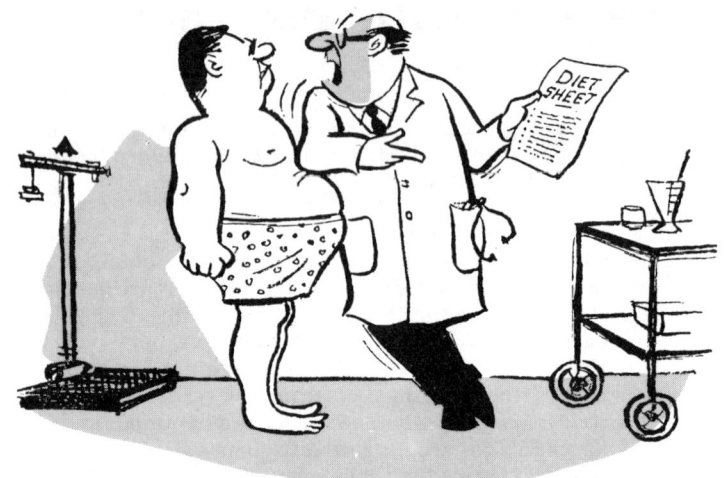

In osteoarthritis diet in itself doesn't matter—except that obesity puts too much strain on weight bearing joints and makes people less active and less mobile

does not cause loss of general health and does not affect one's insurance policy. It is not due to "acids in the system", viruses, or bacteria and is not caused or cured by any particular foodstuffs or drinks. Overweight people on the whole suffer more from it than the slim, however, nobody is immune.

At the menopause

One variety of osteoarthrosis occurs in women around the time of the menopause causing aches in finger tips, thumbs, knees, neck, and elsewhere. Fortunately it tends to abate some years later. This variety, common in women in western civilisation, is relatively rare in certain native African communities but they tend to suffer rather more from osteoarthrosis from local injuries to bone and joint.

Rheumatoid arthritis

Rheumatoid arthritis is an entirely different disorder from osteoarthrosis. Here patients of any age may be affected from the age of 2 years onwards. Most patients are women and most start their illness between the ages of 30 and 50. In Britain it affects around two people in a 100 but is much less common than osteoarthrosis.

What causes it and why certain people get it is unknown. It rarely occurs in several members of one family. Unlike osteoarthrosis it is an inflammatory disease with swelling of the joints and soft tissues round the joints and a feeling of illness, sometimes with fever and often with anaemia, that patients with osteoarthrosis do not experience.

The joints affected are the fingers (but not the joints at the ends of the fingers affected so often in osteoarthrosis, the so called Heberden's nodes after the British physician who wrote about them in the 18th century), thumbs, wrists, elbows, shoulders, bases of the toes, feet, ankles, knees, hips, and jaws. All of these joints may be affected or only a few but they tend to be involved symmetrically on each side. The disease may stop and start, come and go, fizzle out completely, or progress relentlessly. It is an extraordinarily variable disorder which can affect one or two, or almost all the joints in the body for a few days, a few weeks, months, years, and sometimes for ever.

Future unpredictable

There is no certain way of predicting what will happen in any patient. This is what depresses patients so much—they see the disease as unpredictable and possibly never ending, which often produces overtones of anxiety and depression. The joints, initially inflamed and swollen, may become less so but stiffness and deformity may persist and progress so that joints will not go through their full range of movement.

Four unpleasant symptoms

The quartet of nastiness affecting these joints is a variable mixture of **pain, swelling, tenderness**, and **stiffness**. These in turn may cause considerable disability and sometimes crippling deformity but it must be re-emphasised that the disease can and does often settle down and only a minority of patients progress to complete crippling. Only a minority recover completely, however, most continuing to show some change in some joints for many years and often permanently. Happily the spine is seldom affected and the neck only in severe cases.

Other types of polyarthritis

Polyarthritis is a term used for any inflammatory condition of several or many joints. The best known is rheumatoid arthritis, described above but there are many other types. Some, such as the disorder called **ankylosing spondylitis** affects principally the spine, mostly in young men and usually starting between the ages of 17 and 27. Some are associated with psoriasis (a chronic skin condition) some with certain types of colitis. Others, such as the variety that occurs with German measles (rubella), last usually only a few days and recover completely. To make the diagnosis of any form of polyarthritis there must be signs of swelling and tenderness in several joints. Pain in a joint or joints is not enough.

Rheumatic fever—a disappearing disease

Rheumatic fever used to be a most unpleasant disease as it was most common in children under the age of 16 and often affected the heart permanently. Happily it is now rare in this country. A similar disease called **systemic lupus erythematosus** has become rather more common in the last 30 years but this is largely because doctors are more aware of its existence and are diagnosing it more often since the discovery of certain diagnostic blood tests.

Gout—nothing to joke about

Gout is caused by too much uric acid in the body, either because the patient makes too much, eliminates too little through the kidney, or does both. It often runs in families, men

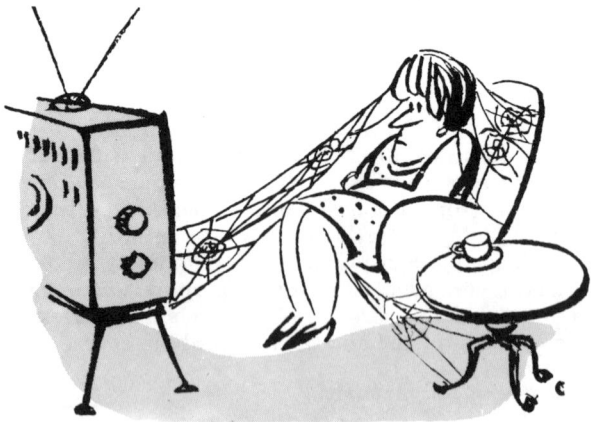

Take sufficient rest but don't fall into the trap of sitting too long in one position

being affected far more often than women, usually when past middle age.

Gout differs from other types of acute arthritis in being more acutely painful. It is said: "put a cord around the toe, tighten it twice and that is arthritis, tighten it several times more, that is gout!" This acutely painful sudden inflammation usually affects only one joint and that is most often the big toe with a red shininess of the skin stretched tight by the swelling and inflammation so that the joint looks like a very painful tomato.

Gout often comes on at night and may be precipitated by too much food or alcohol or too much exercise. In fact, too much of anything or everything. A starvation diet may precipitate it, so excessive virtue may be as productive of attacks as excessive vice! Changes of routine are often responsible so gout is more common in men on holidays or business tours away from home. The acute inflammation is due to crystals of urate precipitating out from the blood into joint tissues. Many useful drugs are now available for its prevention and treatment and gout is now a controllable and largely preventable disease.

Backache—a common problem

Backaches are among the commonest disabilities affecting mankind and cause more time off work than all other rheuma-

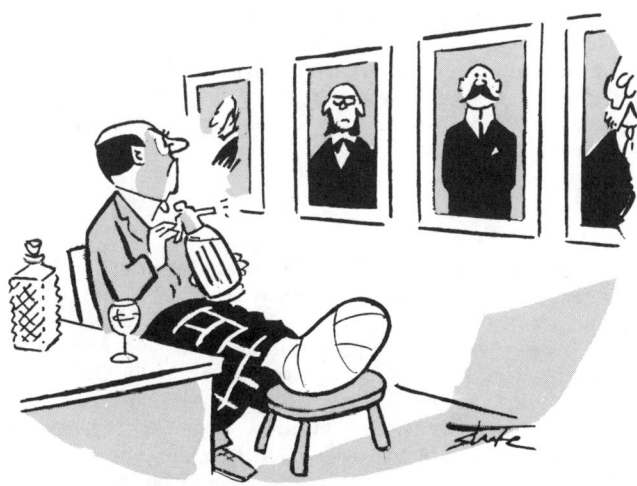

Gout is often inherited and not caused by alcohol, although an attack may be triggered off by overdoing it

tic disorders. The spine is a most elaborate column of 24 vertebrae sitting one on top of another, based on a large bony bowl—the pelvis—and topped by the skull. Between the vertebrae are the discs, elastic cartilages or cushions, acting as shock absorbers. Around them are ligaments and capsules which as they contain many nerve endings are very sensitive to pressure, tears, and stretching. At the back are small joints between adjacent vertebrae; these joints may be affected by some forms of arthritis.

The spine is built for stability and mobility. Running through a tunnel in it (the vertebral canal) is the spinal cord, a direct extension of sensitive nervous tissue from the brain down to the lumbar region, giving out nerves between each vertebra to the body at different levels and to the arms and legs. It is no great wonder that backaches are common and that the exact cause is uncertain, many diagnoses being inspired guesses based on probabilities rather than certainties.

Lumbago is just another way of saying "lumbar (low) backache". **Sciatica** is a term often used loosely by the sufferer to indicate a pain running down the leg from the back or buttock; used scientifically it means pain in the distribution of the sciatic nerve due to involvement of that nerve by some disease process and manifested by the finding of certain changes on examination of the central nervous system. The commonest cause of true sciatica is probably pressure on the nerve root by a ruptured intervertebral disc protruding from the spinal column but there are many other causes. But low backaches may extend into leg or thigh without sciatic root pressure for pains are often referred downwards from many disorders of the lumbar spine.

Causes and effects

The commoner causes of low backache are fatigue; back strain; overwork; bad chairs; bad posture at work, at home or in the car; and even mental depression, for a mild backache may become more severe in the face of anxiety, worry, and particularly depression. Ligaments may be torn or strained by sudden exertions, particularly lifting weights with the spine bent, sudden twisting movements, or falls. Few backaches do not respond to rest, supports, or pain killing medicines but they may take days, weeks, and sometimes months to do so. Very few patients need to have surgery. Time, rest, and avoidance of strain heal most.

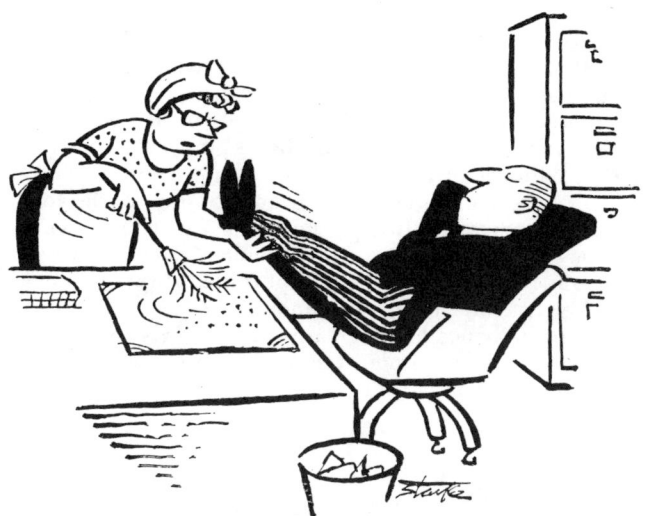

Slouching in a comfy chair may be pleasant, but it makes your back vulnerable to stresses and strains

Most people with chronic backaches prefer to sleep on a firm mattress, often with a board beneath it. A sagging mattress will aggravate most low backaches and a firm support beneath the spine and buttocks may help considerably. A continental quilt or duvet does not have to be tucked in, is easy to manipulate, and saves bed making, which often aggravates backaches. If you are stuck with seats at home, in the office, or car that do not properly support the small of the back, a small cushion or other support is useful to hold the spine upright and prevent the "painful slouching" position. Lifting weights with the spine bent often aggravates backaches. It is best to kneel or squat so that the spine is held straight on these occasions. Supports and corsets are useful in the acute painful stages but most patients prefer to discard them when the acute symptoms abate.

Osteoarthrosis of the lumbar spine, though quite common in later life, is seldom severe or incapacitating and **scoliosis,** or the crooked (sideways bent) spine, is rarely a cause of severe backache. As women age their spinal vertebrae become somewhat lighter in texture and less firm after the menopause. This so called **osteoporosis** may become acutely painful if one of

21

the vertebral bodies becomes squashed—that is develops a crush fracture, the bone becoming compressed. The pain may be slight or severe but even if agonising usually settles down within two or three weeks after bed rest.

Vertebrae may sometimes be displaced on each other, a kind of dislocation called **spondylolisthesis** but as often as not this is either painless or causes little discomfort and it is often a surprise to see appreciable changes in the x-rays of the spine in a patient who has had little or no discomfort whatsoever.

This is true throughout the whole field of rheumatic disease. It isn't what the x-ray looks like that is important but what the joints feel like and how they function. X-rays tell you what goes on in the bones but the pains usually arise elsewhere in the soft tissues which in most cases do not show on x-rays.

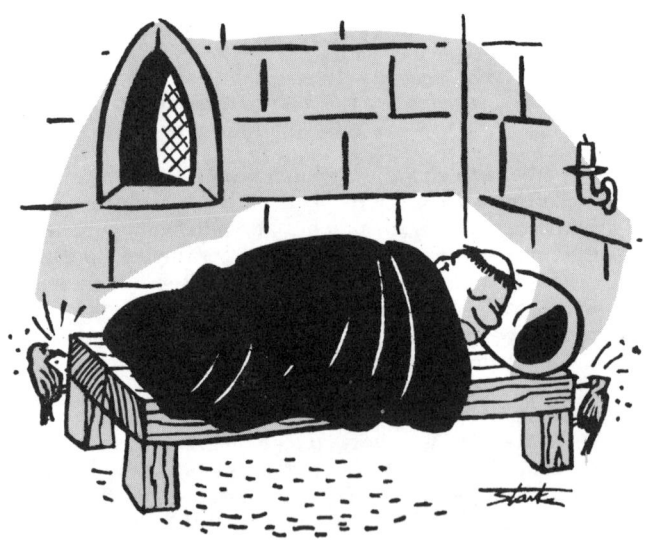

Rest in bed with a board under the mattress is helpful for lumbago

Things that help

—and things that don't

A number of patent medicines which purport to help rheumatic sufferers, can be bought without prescription across the counter. Many do, as they contain a simple painkilling drug such as aspirin or paracetamol but the addition of large numbers of other ingredients often makes little difference. Contrary to many people's belief, purgatives and laxatives do not directly affect the rheumatic condition and do not have any antirheumatic properties. The same can be said of a large number of so called health foods and herbal products.

Aspirin, the great standby in every home, takes moderate and mild pains away and eases the more severe ones in doses of two or three tablets two or three times a day. In bigger doses than this, at regular intervals under your doctor's instruction,

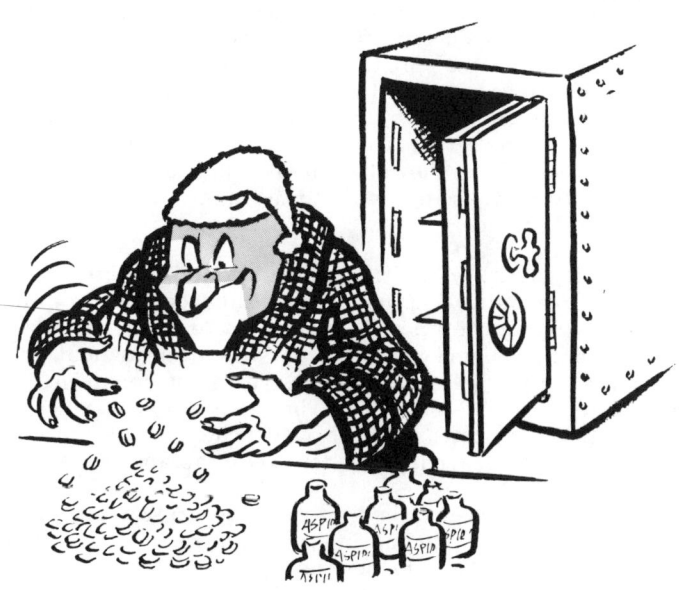

Aspirin remains your most valuable drug

it can reduce inflammation and be useful in many different types of arthritis. Aspirin comes in many forms and combinations and has held its place in public esteem since it was introduced in 1899 but it can cause indigestion and at high doses deafness and ringing in the ears. A few people are allergic to it and develop asthma.

Ibuprofen also relieves pain and damps down inflammation. It can be bought over the counter without prescription and is a useful alternative to aspirin; but like aspirin it may cause stomach upsets.

Paracetamol, like aspirin, reduces pain and fever but it does not reduce inflammation—it is a straightforward pain killer, as is pentazocine, codeine, and dihydrocodeine.

Codeine is constipating and not a strong pain killer; dihydrocodeine is stronger, somewhat mentally relaxing, and slightly constipating.

Cortisone, and cortisone-like drugs are very effective anti-inflammatory drugs, reducing inflammatory swelling and relieving pain in rheumatoid and similar forms of arthritis but usually in a dose that produces many other unwanted side effects. They have to be used very carefully, critically, and in low dosage in this disease, though they are very helpful in other usually more serious disorders. Injected into an inflamed but not infected joint they often help considerably as they do in tennis elbow when injected into the painful area and into stiff, painful shoulders.

Gold salts given by injection and **d-penicillamine** (a by product of penicillin) and the antimalarial drugs, **chloroquin** and **hydroxychloroquin** given by mouth are useful drugs but patients must be under close observation throughout the prolonged period (often of several years) of treatment as unwanted side effects may occur. These drugs have no place in the treatment of osteoarthrosis, backaches, or similar disorders; their only place is in the long term therapy of rheumatoid arthritis.

Many new antirheumatic drugs are appearing every year, relieving pain and reducing inflammation in the joints and inflamed tissues. They do not, however, actively cure any rheumatic disease but by suppressing pain, swelling, and tenderness make life more liveable for the patient. They may

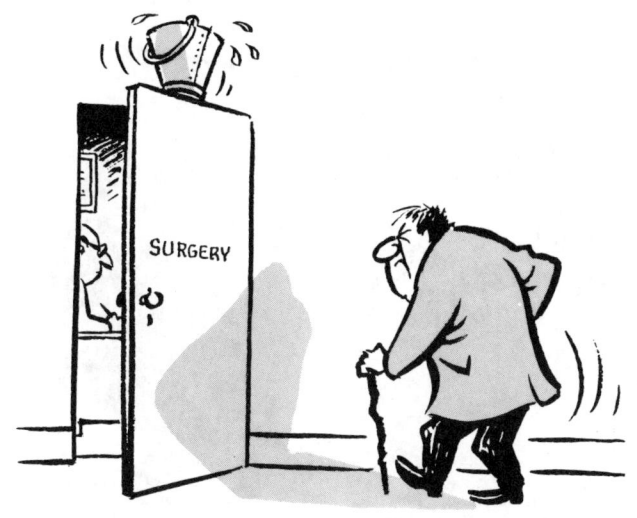

Many new drugs are helpful. They may not cure your rheumatism but they certainly damp things down and "put the fire out"

not put out the fire but they certainly damp it down and encourage it to go out.

Other methods of treatment

Physical methods of treatment—heat, exercises, assisted movements, and exercises and movements in water have been popular since Roman times. Massage and manipulation help many patients but not all and some patients are made worse by vigorous manipulation and movements. Cold (ice) packs and cold applications and sprays are also popular. They produce an "after glow" which often helps the patient considerably.

Don't put your faith in magic

There is no real evidence that copper bangles, nutmegs, new potatoes, or any other magic charms worn or held in the pocket have any effect on any form of arthritis. Similarly, apart from gout and a few rare arthritic disorders, there is little evidence that diet affects any arthritic process. There are, however, two exceptions—gout may be precipitated by rich foods and drinks and, in any form of arthritis where weight bearing joints are affected, overweight is a great handicap. People are healthier

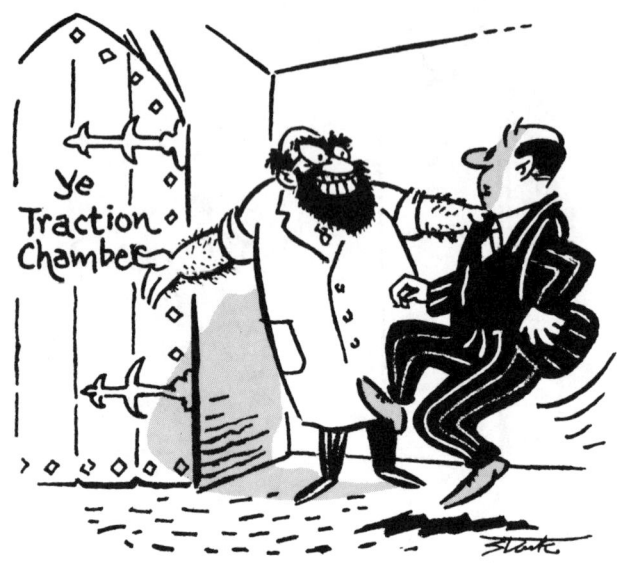

Traction simply means gently stretching the spine by mechanical means

when slim and the rheumatic sufferer very definitely so. Obesity should be avoided in any arthritic disorder and carbohydrates (sugar, bread, pastries, and rice, etc) resisted. Otherwise there is little evidence that any diet affects osteoarthrosis or rheumatoid arthritis.

What about acupuncture?

Acupuncture may relieve pain but does not cure the underlying condition and if all other treatment and medicines are stopped when it is given the patient may become much worse.

What about cold and damp?

Most sufferers from any form of rheumatism will tell you that cold and damp make their rheumatism worse. This is half true. These factors do not make the disease itself worse but they certainly make the pains and aches more acute. Whether due to rheumatism, arthritis, or any other disorder, changes in barometric pressure may do this. A grey cold miserable day depresses the spirits and lessens tolerance of any chronic pain

Apart from those people who are overweight there is no "special diet" for sufferers from rheumatism

and a warm sunny day often improves the pain and the spirits. A warm house often makes pains easier and a cold one the opposite. Some people are sensitive to cold and obtain considerable relief from backache by wearing a woolly vest or roll-on and a warm scarf for neckache.

Living with rheumatism

Short episodes of pain and stiffness lasting only a few days or weeks may be very distressing at the time but they are soon forgotten. Even a severe prolapsed disc may cause severe backache for weeks or months then disappear completely and be just a remote though still unpleasant memory. Many back-aches and aches in neck, shoulders, arms, and legs may persist, however, and make life a misery. The unfortunate sufferer has to live with (and in spite of) them, which needs much patience

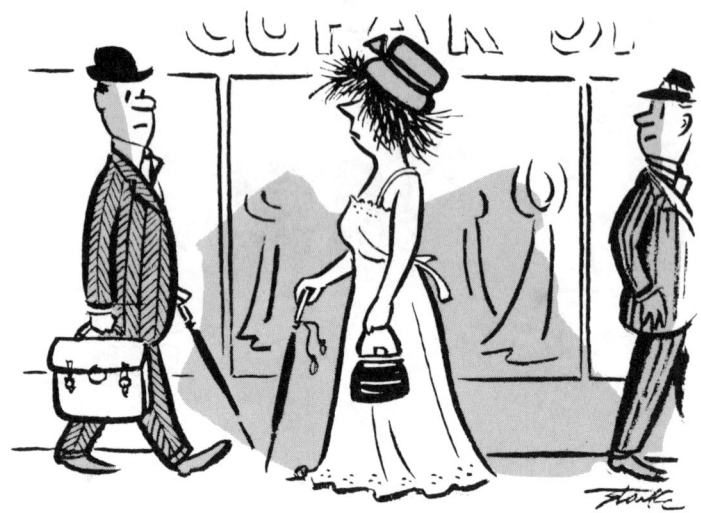

Stiff shoulders make it difficult to dress and do your hair

and fortitude, for constant complaining only puts off other members of the family and sympathy soon runs out.

Helpful aids

What can be done apart from medicines to help chronic aches and pains? Modifications of beds and chairs we have already mentioned. Special gadgets and aids can be used to turn on taps, remove screw tops, pick up objects from the floor, and help many other simple household duties, even putting on socks or stockings. The bathroom and lavatory may be torture chambers for patients with arthritic hips and fitted showers and handles on the side of the bath or small seats in the bath all help.

Each patient, however, has his own problems which have to be solved individually but the local physiotherapy and occupational therapy centre can usually help and the British Red Cross and the Disabled Living Foundation have a great range of gadgets and can inform you where they can be obtained and how much they will cost. Gardening is a great joy to many people who resent the fact that arthritis and rheumatism prevent this activity but again there is a range of gadgets that can help.

Sport and exercise

If feet, knees, ankles, or hips are painfully affected physical exertion involving much walking or running has usually to be restricted considerably. A degree of mobility must be maintained and the joints freely exercised daily, but walking and standing for prolonged periods is OUT. Generally speaking, if exertion causes increased pain or swelling in a joint for two hours or more afterwards, it is too much. Exercise may, however, "tickle up" a joint for an hour or less after which things seem to be rather better for the exertion.

A good general rule is to stick to this one to two hour rule whatever joint is affected. Tennis, squash, golf, badminton may all be played if this rule is not broken. With any arthritis it is wise to travel in a gear lower than the one in which you know you can just manage, so that you do not run on your reserves and become over-fatigued and strain the affected joints. Do everything but do it at your own pace and stop well short of the point of strain or great fatigue. Do it daily but don't overdo it.

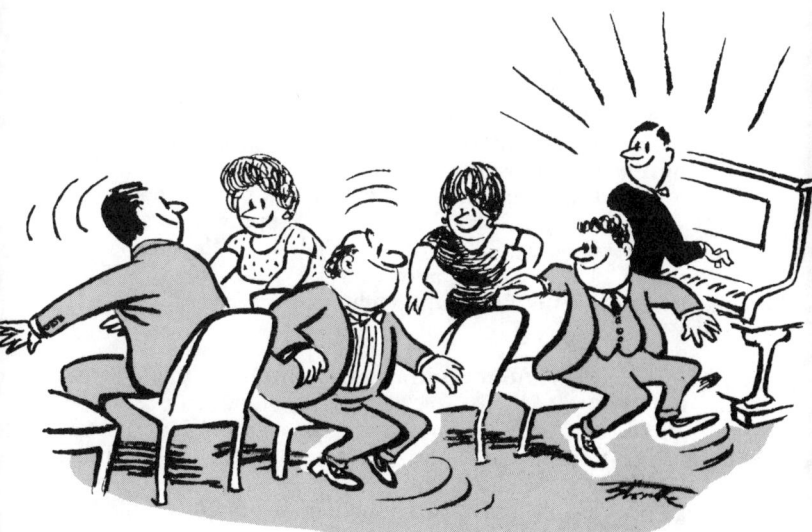

Enjoy yourself but remember to alternate periods of activity with proper periods of rest

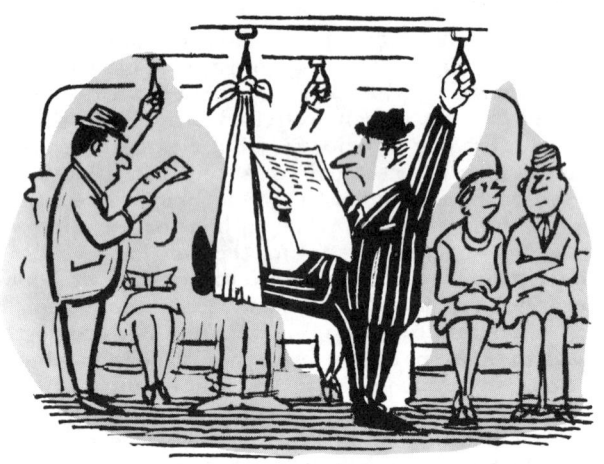

Don't despise active exercises in the home. Going regularly to hospital by public transport for physiotherapy for stiff joints may prove rather awkward!

Organisations that can help you

Central government and local authorities in Great Britain provide many services for disabled people and there are government training centres for the registered disabled. Voluntary organisations such as the **British Red Cross, The Women's Royal Voluntary Service** (W.R.V.S.), **Rotary Clubs** and other organisations help by organising home visits, collecting library books or pensions, shopping, and even providing television sets. The British Red Cross Society is at 9, Grosvenor Crescent, London SW1X 7EJ. (01-235 5454). Branches are listed in local telephone directories.

The Arthritis and Rheumatism Council, 41, Eagle Street, London WC1R 4AR, (01-405 8572) concentrates on research into and education in the rheumatic diseases and deals primarily with doctors rather than the patients direct. They publish useful handbooks which can be purchased by post free of charge (just send a SAE). These include— *Your Home and Your Rheumatism*, and *Marriage, Sex, and Arthritis*. They are an active and busy organisation collecting funds for research into the causes, prevention and treatment of arthritis in over eight hundred branches run by voluntary workers throughout the country.

Arthritis Care, 6 Grosvenor Crescent, London SW1X 7ER (01-235 0902) provides patients with information, advice and practical aids.

The Disabled Living Foundation at 380–384 Harrow Road, London W9 2HU (01-289 6111) has a permanent exhibition of aids and equipment at a special aids centre to help rheumatic patients and provides an information service for them.

The Back Pain Association, 31–33, Park Road, Teddington, Middlesex, TW11 0AB (01-977 5474) aids research and education primarily in the field of backaches in conjunction with the other organisations mentioned above.

The larger local authorities provide a wide range of services for the physically handicapped through their social services and through their health departments.

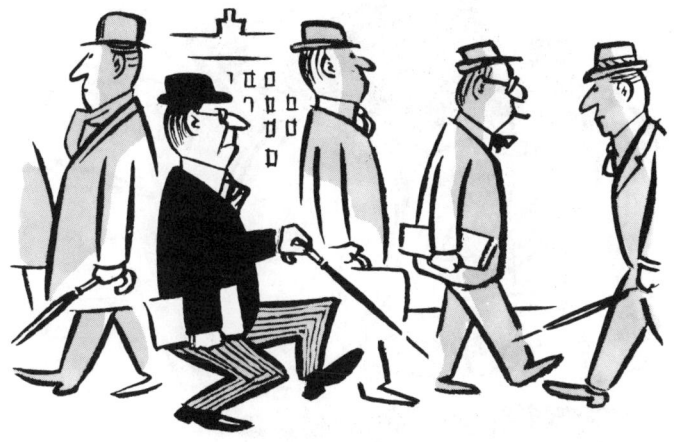

Keep your legs straight in rheumatoid arthritis. It is essential that you never put a pillow under your knees at any time as you may find it difficult to straighten up afterwards

Keeping going

Rheumatic and arthritic sufferers are, however, an independent lot and prefer to keep going under their own steam and usually dislike being registered as Disabled Persons, preferring to struggle on as best they can with what help they can get. No group of patients suffer more pain for longer periods than they do. The rheumatic and arthritic diseases are always a painful nuisance, often disabling but happily rarely fatal or dangerous to life. Nevertheless because they are so common they cause more discomfort to more people than any other group of disorders. Yet most sufferers get on with living as well as they can and rarely complain. Rheumatic Saints and Stoics greatly outnumber Sinners and Complainers!

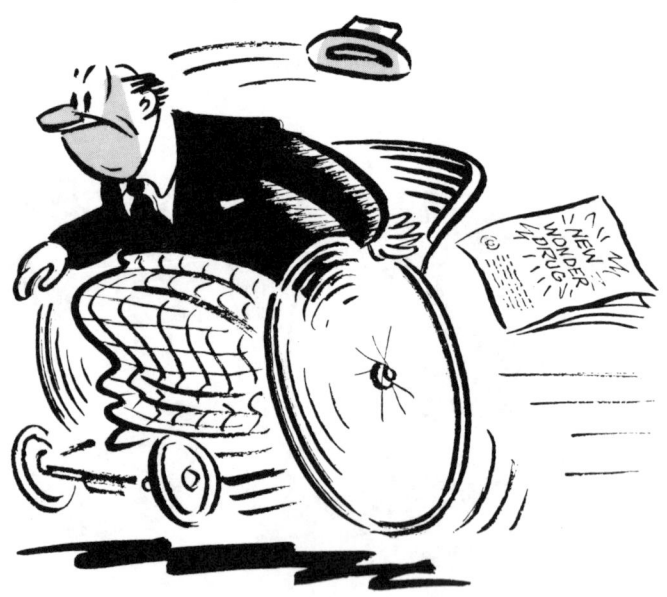

Keep going—but don't rush out after every new cure you read about!

Typeset by Latimer Trend & Company Ltd, Plymouth
Printed in Great Britain by Wm Clowes Ltd, Beccles and London